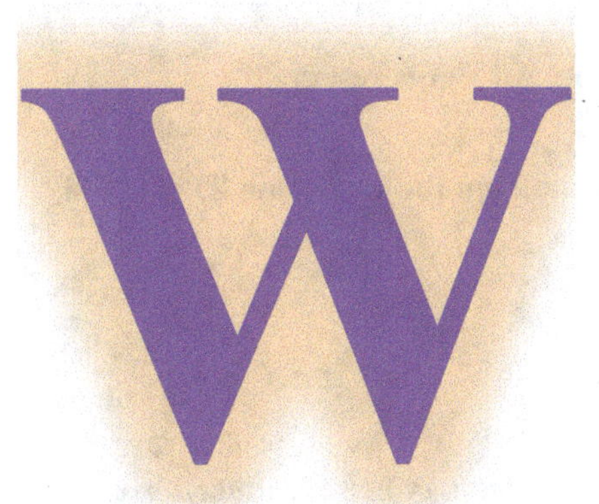

# omen, Permit Yourselves - To be Well…

## By

# ~ Stephanie D. Jones ~

---





## <u>Contact Information:</u>

Stephanie D. Jones

Come Up Higher Ministry LLC

16350 E. Arapahoe Road

Suite 108-255

Foxfield, CO  80016 – 1557

1-682-800-1605

Comeuphigher333@gmail.com

YouTube Channel - www.youtube.com/@CUH333

---

Women, Permit Yourselves ~ To Be Well...

# *TABLE OF CONTENTS*

---

**Women, Permit Yourselves ~ To Be Well…**

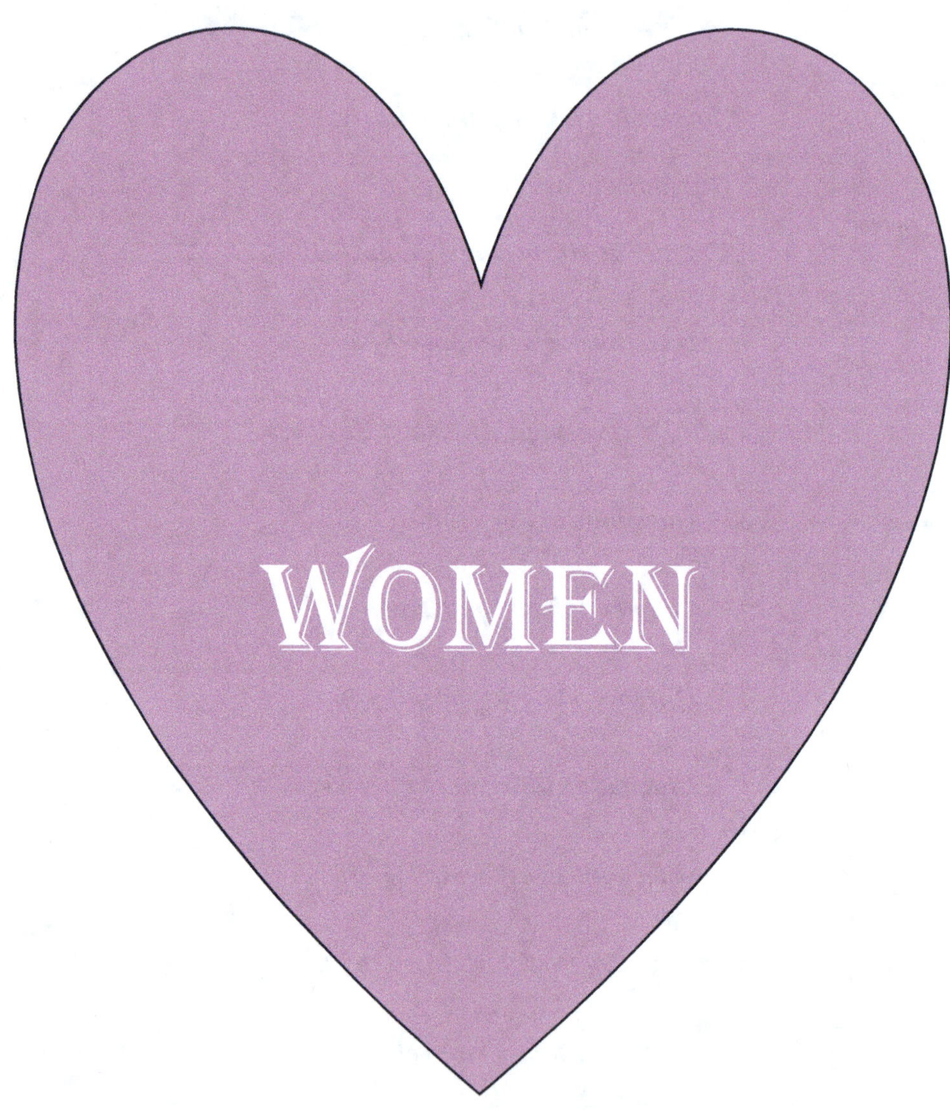


~ 4 ~

**Women, Permit Yourselves ~ To Be Well…**

---

~ The Lord bless and keep you ~

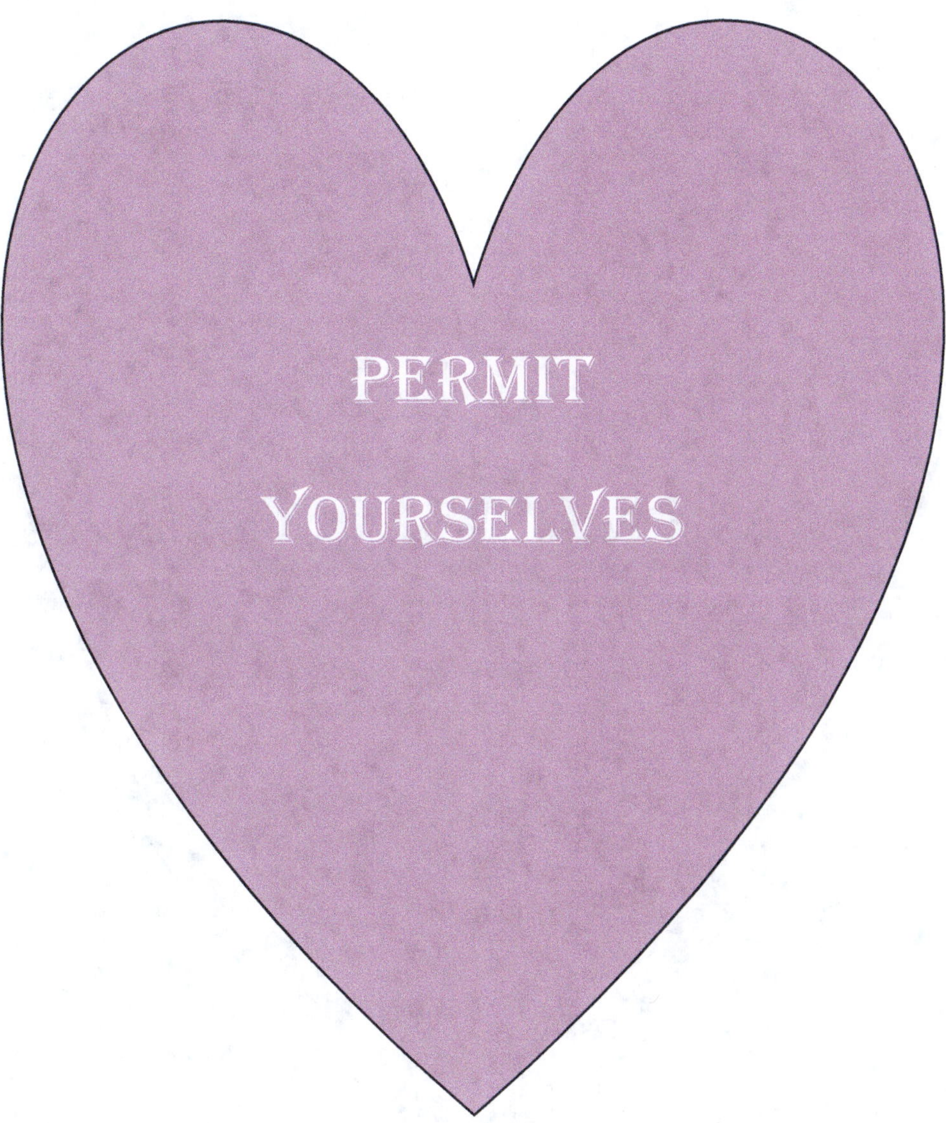
PERMIT

YOURSELVES

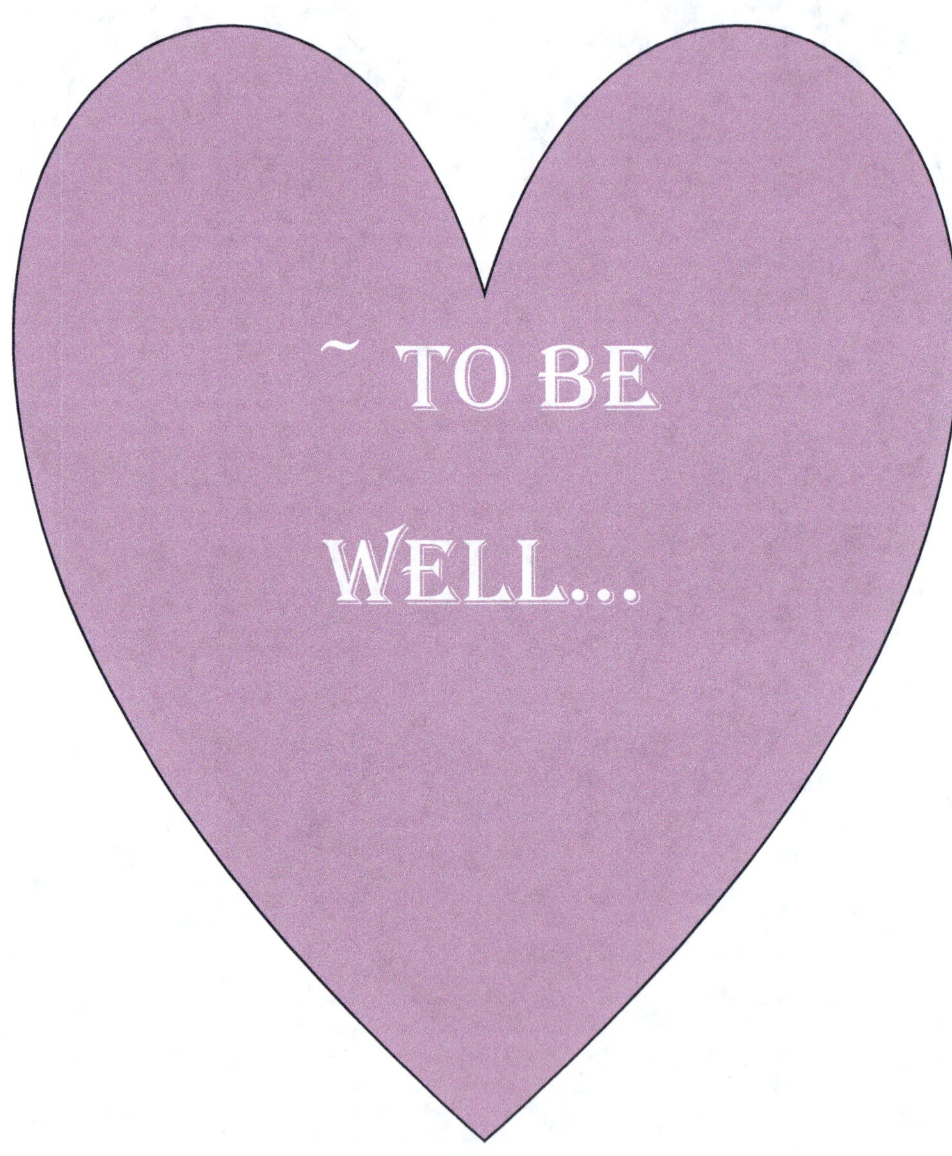
~ TO BE

WELL…

# ~ *Introduction* ~

We live in a world that demands women put everyone before themselves. Often, women's personal needs are ignored, while their voices are disregarded due to the overbearing symphony of the world's expectations, personal obligations, and endless societal bullying. "Women, Permit Yourselves - To be Well" is a heartfelt invitation to reclaim our narratives, prioritize our well-being, and cultivate a space where "wholeness," encompassing mental, physical, and emotional health, takes precedence over everything else.

This book is a personal testimony with an unapologetic tone that gathers women from everywhere to inspire change in our approach to prioritizing ourselves. It acknowledges that we struggle to balance the necessity of self-care while simultaneously showing up in our unmistakable roles as caregivers, professionals, and friends, but unfortunately, and most importantly, not being present for our "Authentic selves!" Somehow, we mistake self-care for a "luxury." Initially, I planned to write this as a "Mission Statement" to myself, but then I realized that someone else may need it as much as I do.  So,

---



I decided to share: Through stories, reflections, and practical insights, I hope to empower us all to break free from the guilt and self-doubt that can stifle our potential to be whole and well. To be very transparent, I am speaking to myself first.

We will cultivate a community where we may thrive in accepting this short message as our permission slip to be well. In doing so, we will commit to prioritizing our needs, embracing our worth, and embarking on a journey toward whole health filled with the care, joy, and wellness we deserve. These pages serve as reminders of new perspectives on the order of priorities.

---

## Chapter 1: *The Weight We Carry*

This book is a heartfelt invitation to women everywhere to embrace health, prioritize self-care, and release the guilt that holds them back. By reclaiming our power, nurturing our bodies and minds, and prioritizing ourselves, we can save our lives and inspire and uplift others. Most women tend to take on the burden of the entire family, including friends and strangers. In doing so, if not mindful, we may gain significant weight and ultimately sacrifice our health/well-being while insisting on caring for those we love. We seem to hold on to fat more, especially around our midsections, where we may carry trauma, unfinished business, or un-birthed purposes and plans, and all these issues are destroying our health. Once we reach the point of "Disease" in our bodies, it often seems impossible to reverse.

As women, many of us feel guilty about our mothers, grandmothers, sisters, daughters, and best friends being fat and unhealthy, so we let ourselves go subconsciously to make others feel better about their miserable situations. When, in all reality, if we held to our truths about how we believe we should look & feel, inside and out, we would be helping to save lives, including our own. By allowing women to take care of themselves and give themselves the same level of care that we provide to others, we will no longer be afraid or ashamed to look at our reflections in the mirror. We will embrace the person staring back at us "wholeheartedly," without shame or fear that we have been unfair to the one person we will spend the rest of our lives dodging if we cannot look into our own eyes.

Near the end of 2020, my mother and I rented a tri-level townhome. Mom is a disabled senior. The place's layout provided bedrooms on the third and basement floors. Either direction included seventeen steps going up, the main floor, and seventeen steps going down. We decided that the third floor would be better for her as she would have natural light and a generous, beautiful master bedroom/bathroom. The basement was just as fantastic: an oversized second master bed and bath, a living area with a quaint television space, and two additional storage rooms. Mom also had access to the laundry room, located right outside her bedroom, as well as two other rooms, and she eventually converted one of them into her office. There was also a full bath in the hallway.

I put a mini refrigerator, microwave, and a mid-sized chest for nonperishable food outside her bedroom to keep her as independent as possible. We eventually used part of the large linen closet in the hallway as a food pantry. In the two-plus years that we lived there, because of her disability, my mother came downstairs only minimally, primarily for doctor's appointments or emergency room visits. Outside those times, I traveled up and down the stairs to take her meals or pick up dishes. I was the only one who cleaned the main floor until we occasionally began using house cleaning services. I was the only one to take out and bring in the garbage can, handle weekly packages/grocery deliveries from the front porch, run all household errands, and pick up the mail. Eventually, I became employed full-time from home, which was a huge blessing because I could be with my mom at home. However, I would work long hours and sometimes manage meals and other daily living responsibilities. There was "No help!"

Unfortunately, I began to pack on weight, mostly around my midsection and upper back. I started to experience physical pain and, in the same year, was diagnosed with Diabetes and Fibromyalgia, on top of the other medical challenges that I was already experiencing. My health had reached a morbid place of "Disease." I was as unhappy as one could be. There was not one area of my body that I felt at ease with. To be honest, I was scared. I felt like I was on my way out.

As for my mom, she is no stranger to challenging work and caring for others. She had six children and raised five; my mom's parents raised her second eldest child in another state. She also survived a divorce after over twenty years of marriage. She spent time caring for their youngest son as a single parent while working full time. She went back to school to be a Nail Technician, only to develop carpal tunnel and require surgery. Sadly, the surgery did not agree with her; my mother was forced to quit the job that she had worked for over five years and went into early retirement. She eventually had to apply for SSDI. Mom also gained weight. With each passing year, she continued to gain weight until her weight eventually spiraled out of control.

**Women, Permit Yourselves ~ To Be Well…**

Along with the heaviness came one health diagnosis after another, one being Colon Cancer, which she survived by the grace of God.

To provide for herself, she became a Host Home Provider. By the year 2020, my mom had spent eleven years caring for an adult disabled woman who became like a family member. The woman was extremely ill when she came to live with my mom. My mother, a Host Home Provider, was approximately sixty-eight at the time, and she managed all the woman's medical needs, took her to appointments, handled all the paperwork, and attended training classes for those eleven years. She also cooked, cleaned, and provided personal care for this person. My mom also participated in activities outside the home for the sake of her client. By the time we all moved into our rental property in October 2020, my mom had checked out both physically and emotionally. She became very ill not long after we moved in.

Ironically, the woman whom my mom cared for and was already suffering from illnesses contracted COVID-19 not too long after we moved in. She was hospitalized and not expected to make it through. One evening, I visited her. She was on a respirator and had not been responsive for days. When I anointed her with Holy oil and began to pray for her, she opened her eyes and watched me. I spoke quietly, reminding her why she needed to live and declaring life over her. I did not stay long. I left immediately after that.

When I stepped outside, I felt led to walk around a wall to avoid disturbing the family walking in my direction. As I turned to go around the dividing wall, I looked down at the most beautiful and impeccably large white feather I have ever seen. There was no wind at all. No birds were anywhere in sight, just a beautiful feather lying on the ground. Was this an "Angel's feather," I wondered. I had often heard that if you see a feather, there is a great possibility that an angel is not far away. It has been over three years since this happened, and I still do not know if I encountered an angel. However, miraculously, the woman I prayed for fully recovered the next day!

After surviving COVID-19, the woman went into a long-term rehabilitation center, and eventually, the agency placed her with another host home provider. I genuinely believe that this was a blessing from God.  As for Mom and me, due to health failure, my mother was physically forced to deal with her medical issues, which meant she would require help. It was my mother's turn to heal and be cared for. The woman she cared for all those years deserved a "Fresh start" with people who could continue the excellent care that she received from my mom when my mother was in the right physical state. At this point, I became my mother's live-in caregiver after others did not work out.

Although she stayed independent and did a lot for herself, I was her legs. I took her to her appointments and emergency room visits. What am I saying here? I am not, in the least, complaining. I am honored and privileged to be there for the woman who gave me life and has loved and cared for me throughout my life. I am simply painting a picture for everyone who, just like my mom, became exhausted from years of taking care of "Everyone else:" Children, a husband, and her disabled client. I, too, had run out of gas. And now I know what it feels like to be "wholly exhausted" and checked out.

Fortunately, our state provided additional help for my mom once we moved into our current residence. I remain her relative caregiver, but she also has a "Homemaker" who comes in five days a week for seven hours. The Homemaker's shift allows me to focus on caring for myself before I must do anything for my mother. Months before my fifty-eighth birthday, this past August 2024, I began working out for thirty minutes; I am up to forty now, at least four times a week. I am now intentional about self-care, something I stopped doing for years.

About two years ago, my mom began taking Ozempic for her diabetes and weight, but once she came to a standstill with weight loss, her doctor switched her prescription to Mounjaro. Instead of throwing away her leftover Ozempic, I decided to try it. It was nearly a two-month supply. During that time, in addition to working out, I lost eighteen pounds and maintained weight loss for about four months. I just learned that I am back in the pre-diabetic range, as I was determined to reverse Diabetes 2. I am finally excited about reaching my health and weight loss goals again! My mom has lost over fifty pounds, had her last knee replacement this past summer, and is determined to have a better quality of life!

## <u>Questions to ask yourself:</u>

1. Are you too **heavy**, either physically, emotionally, or spiritually?

## <u>Questions to ask yourself:</u>

2.  What will you **release** that is not healthy for you?

## <u>Questions to ask yourself:</u>

3.  What will you **adopt** to endorse your new self-discovery of

well-being?

## *Chapter 2: Harboring Trauma*

Too many women are so involved in the well-being of others that we neglect, sometimes consciously, the overbearing conditions in our own lives. Sometimes, these issues become traumas and pain, which settle into our physical bodies, usually in the stomach area. While I am not medically qualified to teach this subject, my experiences may help shed light on it. We must recognize and address the trauma/pain that may eventually lead to a crossroads in one's health. That is what happened to me.

From the time that I started menstruating, when I was twelve years old, I had terrible cramping, nausea/vomiting, and overall feelings of illness accompanying my cycle every month. I delivered my son by C-section when I was twenty-two. At some point, I developed fibroids in my uterus. Early on, my physician told me that they would eventually dissolve. However, the fibroids grew and multiplied outrageously due to my poor eating habits, which included excessive consumption of sugar, carbs, and processed foods. I am sure that my elevated levels of stress and anxiety also significantly impacted how big and how much they multiplied. By the time I was close to thirty, I think, my stomach was protruding, and with each menstrual cycle, I always felt like I was having labor pains. I would have to wear up to four overnight-sized pads to secure myself from any leakage. Every month, I put on a minimum of ten pounds of water weight. I was severely depressed, and my anger was through the roof.

Honestly, I only had one good week every month for years. My son had to put up with my emotional rollercoaster lifestyle his entire childhood. Sadly, he continues to blame me for it to this day.

When I reached around forty-eight years old, the time had come to have them removed. At that point, my Gynecologist suggested that I needed a hysterectomy. Although I was suffering, I was not sure that I was ready to give up, as I was still hoping to find a way to be healed holistically. However, unbeknownst to me, my Gynecologist had grave concerns about my condition and was discussing my case with one of his colleagues, a Gynecological Oncologist, who was adamant that I had Uterine cancer.

So, there I was at a crossroads with my health and clueless as to how severe my medical crisis was. The Gynecological Oncologist sternly warned me that I should start chemo immediately so that I could continue to live for at least another year. She suggested that I would only have six months if I declined to do so. What was baffling was that she had not done a biopsy of my uterus yet and was giving me a "Suspected diagnosis" based on what she had seen in many of her other patients. I will not go into the remainder of that testimony due to time, but I will say that I refused her "Suspected diagnosis" and her chemo.

Instead, I confessed that I did not have cancer, prayed, and stood on the Word of God. I did not sway from what I initially believed or spoke out of my mouth. I held on tightly to my "First confession, which was a direct order that I received from God!"  To sum up my story, the surgeon removed a mass the size of a sixteen-week fetus, four grapefruit-sized fibroids, and, I believe, about eight smaller ones. That's when it became clear to me. That is why I felt like I was having labor pains every time I had my menstrual cycle. That is why I was so miserable and emotional three weeks out of every month for years, and that is why my stomach was protruding, and I would gain so much

water weight each time. Wow! Who knew? Now, that is what I refer to

as "Trauma!" Imagine spending all those decades not knowing what I

was physically carrying inside my body.

Talk about the enemy within. I had no clue.

However, in retrospect, I now understand why I quit everything I

started. It did not matter what it was: a new job, church, gym, or

friendships; I would start with such zeal and excitement, only to lose

interest quickly because I would begin to feel sick, fat, and depressed

beyond my understanding or control. Nevertheless, I was finally ready

to accept what I had done to myself and admitted that I was in trouble. I

had the recommended partial hysterectomy.

At first, following the surgery, I was unable to process that my

menstrual cycle was gone for good. I continued to brace myself for its

hideous impact on my body, mainly because of the incident that followed

my return home from surgery. I was staying with my mom at that time.

One day, she went grocery shopping as I lay on the couch, recovering.

Suddenly, I felt the urge to run to the bathroom. Without warning, clots of blood the size of golf balls rushed out of my body, one after another, until I counted ten of them. As soon as I was able, I called for an ambulance. I remembered that upon discharge from my hysterectomy surgery, the medical staff told me that any sign of bleeding warranted a prompt return.

Once the ambulance arrived, they rushed me back to the hospital, where I received emergency surgery to re-close an incision from within that had opened and collected blood and formed clots. Before the surgery, I cried uncontrollably to the point that the surgeon and the entire staff surrounded me for comfort before putting me under anesthesia. I still get emotional when I think of it; I felt utterly alone at that moment.

Having the emergency surgery did not help me believe that the worst was over. It only magnified, for me, that my menstrual cycle had found a way to avenge itself for my removing my uterus. Or at least that is what my mind was feeding me. I survived the second surgery, but my blood count dropped to six, and the doctors insisted that I have a blood transfusion. Whether I was right or wrong, I decided that a blood transfusion was not a risk that I was willing to take, so I declined. Despite the threats from the five different doctors whom the surgeon sent to tell me that I would indeed "Die" without the procedure, I decided to put all my faith in my God. I prayed before leaving the hospital and believed that God told me to drink significant amounts of water and eat beets often, and that is precisely what I did. Within a month, my blood count was on an incline!

I must admit that I wish I had been more involved in caring for myself long before coming to the place of needing a hysterectomy or the threat of a blood transfusion. If I had been emotionally present for myself, I would have avoided the consequences of the neglect of which I am guilty. Fortunately, I have been able to forgive myself and move toward "New beginnings," where I have decided to reinvent myself by living a life of intentional balance and journaling, a formula God gave me. I will get into that towards the end of this book. Oh, and by the way: The surgeon had biopsies done of the mass and fibroids removed from my uterus, and by the grace of God, "there was no cancer!"

## <u>Questions to ask yourself:</u>

1.  Are you **carrying any trauma** in your stomach? If yes, what

    are they?

## <u>Questions to ask yourself:</u>

2.  Do you need a "**Spiritual hysterectomy,**" so to speak? What needs to be **spiritually or physically** removed?

## <u>Questions to ask yourself:</u>

3. Have you received a **"Suspected diagnosis"** about your health that you know is **a lie**? If so, what is it? What do you intend to **do about it**?

## *Chapter 3: Discovering Unfinished Business*

I am sure that unfinished business, missed opportunities, and unfulfilled purposes, or however you want to refer to them, directly affect our well-being. We experience a lack of fulfillment, shame, and even sorrow. As we confront these truths directly, we can start the process of healing, growth, and self-discovery.

I surrendered my life to Christ in the early part of 1992. Ironically, while I was still very much living a lifestyle of sin, I began to get ideas about writing a spiritual book by the end of 1991. I vividly remember writing down sentences and notes on scrap paper whenever I heard something from within.  Little did I know, then, that it was the Holy Spirit who was feeding me the message. I ate, slept, and lived that book for months before asking Jesus to come into my life and be my Lord and Savior. The book seemed simple, but I had the most difficulty believing God would have me author a book. Therefore, I sat on it for years before the conviction was more than I could bear.

One summer day in 1996, I went into my literal "Prayer closet" at approximately six in the morning. I listened intently as the Holy Spirit downloaded the words to my book, "Come Up Higher!" within me. It was approximately midnight when I walked out, and I had nearly completed one hundred pages. Still, I was not convinced I had heard from God about authoring a book, and I put my draft away for the second time, which turned into even more years.

Eventually, I dusted it off and began to write it again. I even mistakenly shared it with two pastors of a church I had attended briefly, only to have one of them criticize my work without offering any guidance, given that he was a published author. The other pastor began to take excerpts from my book and use them for Sunday sermons. Once again, I put it away and hid behind doubt and fear.

It wasn't until a few years ago, after I received my master's degree in creative writing, that I decided to complete the book and publish it on Amazon. I knew it was not up to par or ready to be published, but I hoped that taking such a drastic step would be the push I desperately needed to make it a reality. I didn't make it available to the public, but I purchased a few copies for my own purposes. I expected to locate a literary agent and have them help me edit and take the book to the next level. I even shared it with a few family members and associates for feedback.  I should never have done that, as it only made me more self-conscious about my work.

I can hardly express to you how much of a burden I felt lifted off me the first time I finished writing it. It was huge. I felt life return to me. I enjoyed being around people again. I began to envision my future again. I do not regret self-publishing it on Amazon before it was ready. I had to get that book out of my head. I had to birth it to realize my purpose as a writer and begin the healing process of my life overall, but especially in my "Birthing location," my stomach area. I can envision how great it will feel once I rewrite it and finally release it for good!

Not too many months ago, in a dream, a voice told me to "Write the book again."  Listen, I don't fully understand why; I have an idea, but I will obey and rewrite "Come Up Higher," as I believe God has called me to do it, and He will make it reach the souls of those who may need to read it. In the meantime, I am birthing other projects while simultaneously fulfilling my primary assignment from God.

God revealed to me, supernaturally, that my purpose is to "inspire a sister, encourage a brother, reach out, and that we all help one another." I believe God has given me a mandate to do all that and "not give up in this race until I see Jesus's blessed face; this is my purpose!" Song by the Pace Sisters: (This is my Purpose, 1992).

## <u>Questions to ask yourself:</u>

1.  Are you **holding on** to any unfinished business/un-birthed

    purpose? If yes, please list them.

## <u>Questions to ask yourself:</u>

2. Do you need to **redo** something to "birth" your purpose? If yes, can you elaborate?

## <u>Questions to ask yourself:</u>

3. If the answer to number 2 is yes, what do you need to redo, or can

   you **tweak, add to, or reduce** it?

## *<u>Chapter 4: The Guilt Trap</u>*

So, why do we often feel guilty about putting ourselves first, which typically accompanies a lack of prioritizing our needs? We constantly measure ourselves against the societal expectations and pressures, "bullying" that push women to neglect themselves in favor of caring for others. By challenging these narratives and permitting ourselves to put our well-being first, we can break free from the guilt trap and step into our power. As the adage goes, "One must first put their oxygen mask on before attempting to do so for another;" Otherwise, one would lose the oxygen necessary to stay alive, at which point, those depending on our help are also at risk of dying.

I have a harrowing story about someone I love immensely. A woman I know was married to her husband for approximately forty years or more. He was around eighty-six, and she was near eighty when he became extremely ill. Sadly, the husband was already enduring different health issues, but once dementia set in, it became challenging for the woman to care for him. Many years prior, the professional couple retired from prestigious jobs, left the East Coast, and returned to the South to settle down and grow old together. They had their final home built to suit their desires, had plenty of money in the bank, and traveled at will.

The wife never missed a hair or nail appointment and was adamant about being up to date with her medical care.  And, whenever she envisioned a fresh look for her home, the contractors were in place, and the Work would be on the way to completion. They were a wonderful couple. You rarely find two people who are so ideally suited for each other. There was an understanding between them. Everyone brought one hundred percent to the table, and nothing was lacking. He treated her like a queen, and she esteemed him as her king.

Eventually, the wife became his full-time caretaker for at least a year because they were uncomfortable with strangers entering their home and often suspected others of wanting what they possessed. During that time, due to dementia, the husband became very territorial of her. Her sacred beauty appointments ended abruptly, as did their morning trips to their favorite fast-food window, where they cherished the breakfast sandwiches, coffee, and the staff, who all knew the couple by their first names.

If she got on the phone, he would scream at the top of his lungs to get her attention. He became physically violent more than once. And he did not want anyone else around. Only when he fell out of bed and onto the floor would he allow her to seek help from the next-door neighbor. She endured this for a year or more before finally taking the advice of concerned family members and friends to allow a professional caregiver to come into the home and help her care for him. By this time, her handwriting skills had diminished; she was very shaky and began to struggle with short-term memory loss.

Sometime during the COVID-19 pandemic, her husband became unresponsive and was admitted to the hospital. When his children arrived out of state, they made it to his bedside just in time to say goodbye, as he did not regain consciousness. I cannot relay all the particulars in this mini book because there are too many. The only reason that I am using this as an example is that after the husband died, the wife was diagnosed with trauma-induced memory loss. She did not have dementia or Alzheimer's disease, according to the test and brain scan that she received.

As I stated earlier, the adage of needing to put on our oxygen masks before helping others put theirs on fits this story precisely. It is quite possible that the woman would not be in her current predicament if she had insisted on putting her health first, continuing what was necessary for "self-care," and allowing professionals to come into their home sooner and give her husband proper care. As I stated, this is an unfortunate story. This beautiful woman, whom I adore, continued to struggle with her short-term memory. After getting lost one day while driving, relatives had to search for her and her vehicle. Fortunately, they located her and got her safely back to her home. Eventually, these family members took her to live with them.

It has been about three years, and the woman still lives with her relatives; sadly, she would never have chosen to do this. I know because she once told me that she planned to live in an assisted living facility if she ever arrived at a place in this life where she could no longer care for herself. However, since she never put it in her Will, her desires will not be fulfilled. Her home, beautifully decorated and worthy of a visit from Martha Stewart, was eventually stripped of its furnishings and is now awaiting sale. At the same time, her Mercedes may have already been sold, and the money will be divided amongst some of her relatives, while the rest will be used to continue her care. The woman and her late husband had built their home from the ground up, and it was nearly paid off when he passed away. As for her, she has been heard saying, repeatedly, "I'll be going back to my house soon; my husband is waiting for me." Sad, right? Yes, really, really, sad.

Nevertheless, I am grateful she is safe, cared for, and with her family. That is all I can hope for at this point. She somehow trusted that her husband's children would be there for her if he transitioned first. She could not have been more wrong. Over these last three years, I have spent hours praying, crying, and hurting for her. However, it quickly became clear to me that I could do nothing except let go and trust in God. Eventually, I began to rehearse the newer saying, "It is what it is."

This is why we must put ourselves first in this race called "Life." There will be an end to something, and we do not want it to take us down with it. Especially if it is not "Our ending." I pray that makes sense to you. No one on this earth will concern themselves with how we need to be cared for as adults more than we will. It is time to prioritize self-care, even if it comes at a cost, if we are not already doing so. I do not care if we must schedule it, cut out some of the children's activities, or say no to everything outside of the mandatory necessities for the next year or until "Self-care" becomes second nature. We must stay on top of our own needs. No negotiations!

# <u>Questions to ask yourself:</u>

1. Have the **feelings of guilt** been keeping you from prioritizing your self-care? If yes, are you being honest with yourself?

## <u>Questions to ask yourself:</u>

2.  Are you forced into making someone else your top priority? If so, can you take any steps to **change the outcome** in your favor?

## <u>Questions to ask yourself:</u>

3. What **steps** must you take before making yourself a priority? Do you need help caring for an aging/ill parent or small children? If yes, **will you seek and receive** the help that you need?

## *Chapter 5: Choosing Life*

I want to take a moment to emphasize the importance of choosing life, "Our own lives. Let us consider the transformative potential of embracing our truths, both within and around us, and their positive impact on our health, happiness, and relationships. I wholeheartedly encourage women to let go of the fear of judgment, jealousy, or rejection and instead embrace a path of wholeness and self-fulfillment.

"My truths:" I want to live in excellent health and weigh my ideal weight, I want to be an accomplished and well sought-after author, I want to be joyfully married and grow old with my husband, I want a great deal of land and to build our dream home and my mom's dream home attached to ours. I would love for my in-laws to build a house on that land. I will invite like-minded family members and friends, as well as strangers who will become like family, and share our vision of "living on that land" with them. I envision caring for our elderly, youth, and each other on that land. I see lots of food and beautiful gardens emerging from the earth on that land. Believe me when I say there is so much more, but I will save them for another time.

My point is that I have desires and goals that are my truths, and I deserve to see them all come to fruition. We all deserve to see our dreams and truths come to life in our lives. They are our "Truths!" It will never matter who disagrees with our truths or who is angry or jealous about what we want for our own lives or families. And, until we birth these truths out of our bodies, we will continue to feel unfulfilled, or worse, we may begin to rot from within. Our rot may become a "Disease" in our bodies, making it extremely difficult to accomplish our truths or God-given mandates. That's right! We do not answer to man. We will respond to God, "Creator of all," when we face Him, and He asks us, "What did you do with what I gave you?"

Please check out this parable that Jesus shared with His Disciples:

**Matthew 25:14-30 – The Parable of the Ten Talents (NKJV) 14**

> **"For the kingdom of heaven is like a man traveling to a far country, who called his servants and delivered his goods to them. 15 And to one he gave five talents, to another two, and to another one, to each according to his own ability; and immediately he went on a journey.**

16 Then, he, who had received the five talents, traded with them and made another five talents. 17 And likewise, he who had received two gained two more also. 18 But he who had received one went and dug in the ground and hid his Lord's money. 19 After a long time, the Lord of those servants came and settled accounts with them.

20 "So he who had received five talents came and brought five other talents, saying, 'Lord, you delivered to me five talents; look, I have gained five more talents besides them.' 21 His lord said to him, 'Well done, good and faithful servant; you were faithful over a few things, I will make you ruler over many things. Enter into the joy of your Lord.' 22 He also who had received two talents came and said, 'Lord, you delivered to me two talents; look, I have gained two more talents besides them.' 23 His Lord said to him, 'Well done, good and faithful servant; you have been faithful over a few

things, I will make you ruler over many things. Enter into the joy of your Lord.'

24 "Then he who had received the one talent came and said, 'Lord, I knew you to be a hard man, reaping where you have not sown, and gathering where you have not scattered seed. 25 And I was afraid and went and hid your talent in the ground. Look, there you have what is yours.'

26 "But his Lord answered and said to him, 'You wicked and lazy servant, you knew that I reap where I have not sown and gather where I have not scattered seed. 27 So you ought to have deposited my money with the bankers, and at my coming, I would have received back my own with interest. 28 So take the talent from him and give it to him who has ten talents.

29 'For to everyone who has, more will be given, and he will have abundance; but from him who does not have, even what he has will be taken away. 30 And cast the unprofitable servant into the outer darkness. There will be

---



**weeping and gnashing of teeth.' (This entire passage is taken from the Holy Bible, NKJV).**

Wow, I do not know about you, but that parable grabs my heart whenever I read it. Please do not think for a moment that I am trying to scare anyone, including myself. All I am attempting to do is to remind those of us who want to fulfill the call of God on our lives or fulfill our "truths" that we will someday have to produce to the King of Kings and Lord of Lords what we have accomplished while here on earth.  In the meantime, consider this: when we look ourselves in the eye, we are checking in with our current reality, and our soul is asking, at that moment, "Are you working towards your truth?"

---

## <u>Questions to ask yourself:</u>

1. What are your **truths**? Are you, at the very least, working toward fulfilling them?

## <u>Questions to ask yourself:</u>

2.  Have you multiplied your **God-given talents** or buried them?

What are they?

## <u>Questions to ask yourself:</u>

3.  Is your soul content with your **choices**?  If not, why?

## *Chapter 6: The Power of Authenticity*

In this concluding chapter, let us celebrate our willingness to make ourselves a priority. And I assure you that I do not make light of the fact that it will take all our strength and courage to fulfill our journey to wholeness. We acknowledge that not everyone will understand or support our choices, but that those willing to join us on this journey are the ones who truly matter. Women are even more empowered when we surround ourselves with a supportive community and release those who hinder our progress. It is time to choose life and fill our cups to overflow with the good things that await us on the path of self-love and self-discovery. Together, let us embark on this journey of embracing wholeness and self-care with impeccable and intentional care.

Once on the road back to our authentic selves, it does not matter who becomes jealous, angry, or walks away from us because we choose to be healthy inside and out; we will always know where they are. Again, it is time to decide. We can choose to follow those who refuse to make the necessary changes in their lives and for their health because, at the end of the day, "their goal is to keep us as unhealthy as they are." Or, again, we can choose life! I trust that you share my sentiment in wanting to "Live!" Furthermore: "Those who are willing to follow, join, or lead on this path of 'Self-care to Wholeness,' are welcome. Those who choose to hinder may kindly have a seat in the "Back rows of our lives." Now, that is the way to be authentic!

Earlier, at the end of chapter two, I mentioned how I went back to living my life based on a formula given to me by God. In conclusion, I would love to share this enormous revelation and gift I received from Him, who loves us unconditionally.

So, decades ago, I was a single parent raising my son. One day, I was on the treadmill. I was enjoying myself. During those times, I was extremely close to God and would hear His still, small voice very clearly and regularly, and I would seldom misinterpret it. While moving briskly on the machine, I profoundly listened to the voice of God tell me that I would live a balanced and successful life if I did these four things – daily: "Spiritual, Work, Exercise, and Play." Can you believe it? Well, I took this to heart, and let me tell you, my life began to smooth out, and things started falling into place for my son and me.

I immediately put our home on a strict schedule and adhered to it without deviation. I was disciplined and focused on obeying God's words, reaping the benefits of my obedience, and being open and willing to hear and receive guidance and revelation from Him. Journaling was already a daily part of my life and a "must" for me, as it tracks years of testimonies, trials, tribulations, accomplishments, and more, which results in growth, spiritual progress/promotions, and healing. I also fasted once a week and did an extensive fast at the beginning of each new year on behalf of my entire family and myself. Fasting regularly was one of the reasons I was able to hear God's voice so clearly.

My schedule consisted of an early wake-up at 4:45 am, where I spent the first fruits of my day with God through prayer, praise/worship, meditation, and reading the Bible; this was my "**Spiritual**." I devoted time to my job; this was my "**Work**." I would walk in the park or on the treadmill and do dance aerobics at home for an hour; this was my "**Exercise**." Finally, my son and I would have dinner, do his homework, and get clothes ready for the next day. Then, it was downtime, my "**Play**," usually something funny on television back then. Of course, our schedule also consisted of house chores, which I did on Thursdays, so I had no chores for the weekends when Work ended on Fridays. I designated a day solely for laundry, as our schedule also included reading the Bible at night, journaling my day, an eight pm bedtime for my little guy, and a sharp ten pm lights out for me. Despite my monthly menstrual blues, those were some of the best times of our lives. I thrive on organization and order, among other things.

I cannot tell you when I wandered off that path, but at some point, I became distracted and stopped following my God-given formula for balance and success. If I am correct, it was a man. In retrospect, most of the times that I got off course were because I was entertaining distractions, which usually showed up in the form of a person, to be quite honest. What a waste of my time, my life, my journey.

Nevertheless, I am happy to report that I am "fighting hell" to get back on my journey to live a successful life through my God-given formula of "Balance." I would love to tell you that it is an easy jump back, but that would not be honest. In all transparency, this has been one of the hardest things for me to do at this point in my life. It is truly one of my greatest battles, and that's because the enemy (Satan) knows that if he can keep me from achieving my goal of living in the manner that God showed me will be favorable, then I will not have a "Balanced and successful life. However, because God gave it to me, I know with every fiber of my being that I cannot go wrong once I get there! It is a "Fail-proof" plan, and I have lived it, walked it out, and managed to do so for a long time. So, I know that it works. Again, I remember how, despite my horrible menstrual cycles, my life felt right. I experienced the feeling of living intentionally, with God-given instructions and purpose, which was utterly fulfilling, and I yearn for that again.

This time around, I will be able to enjoy my life so much more since I no longer have those hideous monthly menstrual cycles. Now that I am back to focusing on self-care and committed to living a balanced life, along with daily journaling and weekly fasting, I am confident that everything will fall into place again. Having said all that, I invite you to join me on this newfound and joyful journey of "Self-care to Wholeness" and a balanced life through daily journaling and implementing four key steps into our everyday schedules. I have also created a "Balance through Journaling" journal to help us reinvent ourselves, which I trust will serve as an excellent jump-start to this new lifestyle. I pray you will agree. Let me leave you with this:  If you refuse to permit yourself, my fellow women, then allow me:  "Sister, I give you permission to be well..."

## **<u>Questions to ask yourself:</u>**

1.  Are you willing to make **yourself a priority**?  Why?

## <u>Questions to ask yourself:</u>

2.  Have you decided to **choose life**?  Why?

## <u>Questions to ask yourself:</u>

3. Are you ready to live a **balanced life** through a "Fail-proof

   "Formula?  Why?

Well, friends, that's all I have for now. I truly hope this short read has blessed you as much as it has me. I cried while editing this. I allowed myself to listen to it through "Read Aloud," at a slower to medium speed, which captures my tone perfectly. I found myself processing some of my hidden traumas, pain, and unfinished business, among other things. I pray this book will personally touch your heart the same way, so that healing may begin.

There's one last thing that I must do before I go: I must share a prayer of salvation with you. Check out this brief scripture from Romans 10:9 (NKJV):

"That if you confess with your mouth the Lord Jesus and believe in your heart that God has raised Him from the dead, you will be saved."

If you have never invited Jesus into your heart to be the Lord and Savior of your life or would like to return to Christ, please say the prayer on the following page…

---

Women, Permit Yourselves ~ To Be Well...

*Dear Lord Jesus,*

*I repent of all my sin, wrath, rebellion, and disobedience and ask for your forgiveness. I confess that you are Lord and the Son of the Living God.  Will you please come into my heart and be my Lord and Savior? I ask this in your name, Jesus, amen.*

*If you have prayed this prayer, the angels are celebrating your salvation at this very moment (Luke 15:10). Next, ask Father God, in the name of Jesus, to fill you with His Holy Spirit! That's it, you are on your way! The Holy Spirit will guide you from here to where you will fellowship and any changes you may need to make "To please the Lord." Enjoy your new walk and relationship with God: The Father, Son, and Holy Spirit.*

*PS: I love you!*

*~ Stephanie D. Jones ~*

---

## *About the Author*

*Who is Stephanie Jones? I am a new author whose greater purpose*

*is to encourage others. I desire to help others along their spiritual*

*journey of purpose and living "Intentionally" for God.  I*

*"Supernaturally" received an excerpt from the song "This is my*

*Purpose," by the Pace Sisters, many years ago: "To inspire*

*a sister, encourage a brother; to reach out and help one another. This*

*is my Purpose."   I considered that encounter to be my "Mandate*

*from God!"*

*I enjoy taking a more practical approach to writing, with an*

*unapologetic tone of my love for God. I will always strive to keep my*

*authenticity as my balance and foundation.  I will "always" share*

*personal and true stories about my life in the hopes that others will*

*be able to relate to me and realize that they are not alone, and that*

*God does take what was meant for harm and make it work together*

*for good to those who love Him and are the called according to His*

*purpose (Romans 8:28).*

*While I have not yet arrived, I thrive on sharing that I am consistently working towards moving from glory to glory with a zeal to live out what I write about and invite others to join me. I am transparent and honest. I have a healthy reverence for God and have developed a genuine, loving relationship with Him. I confess that every time I work on a spiritual project, it brings me closer to God. I am clear: I am doing this for His Kingdom, His children. May we never forget: "Only what we do for God will last" (C.T. Studd, Only One Life, exact year unknown).*

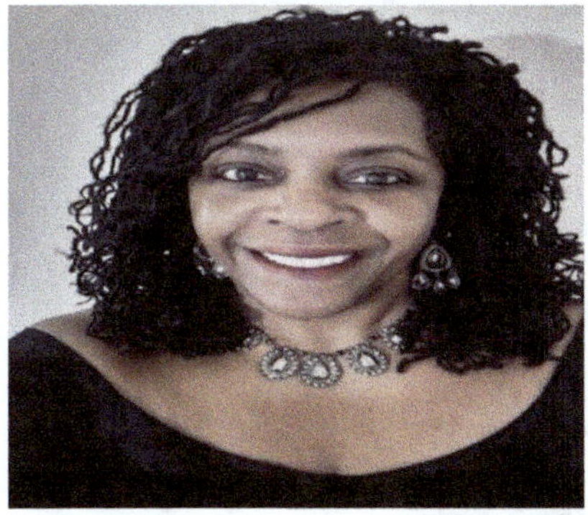

*~ Stephanie D. Jones ~*

# ♥ NOTES ♥

**Women, Permit Yourselves ~ To Be Well…**

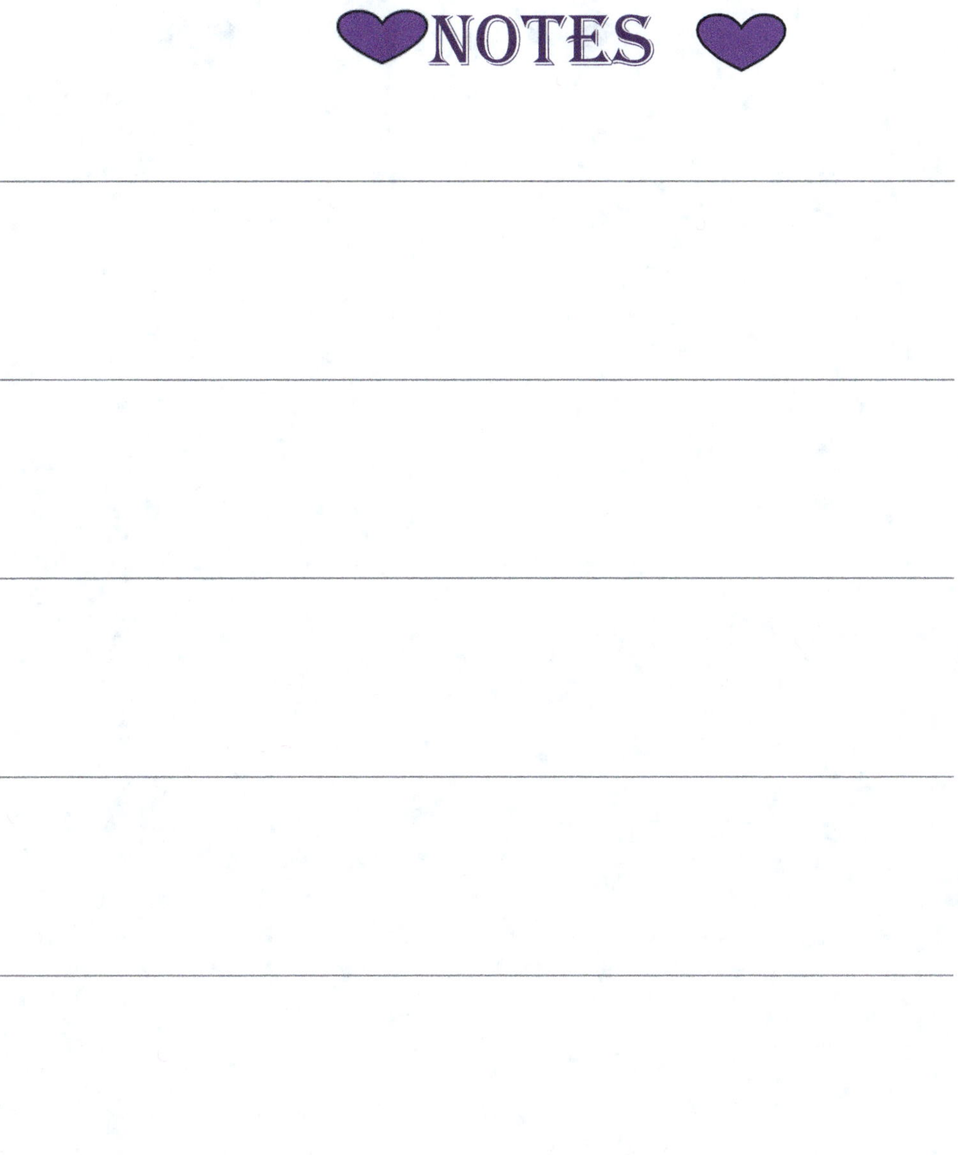

# ♥ NOTES ♥

**Women, Permit Yourselves ~ To Be Well…**

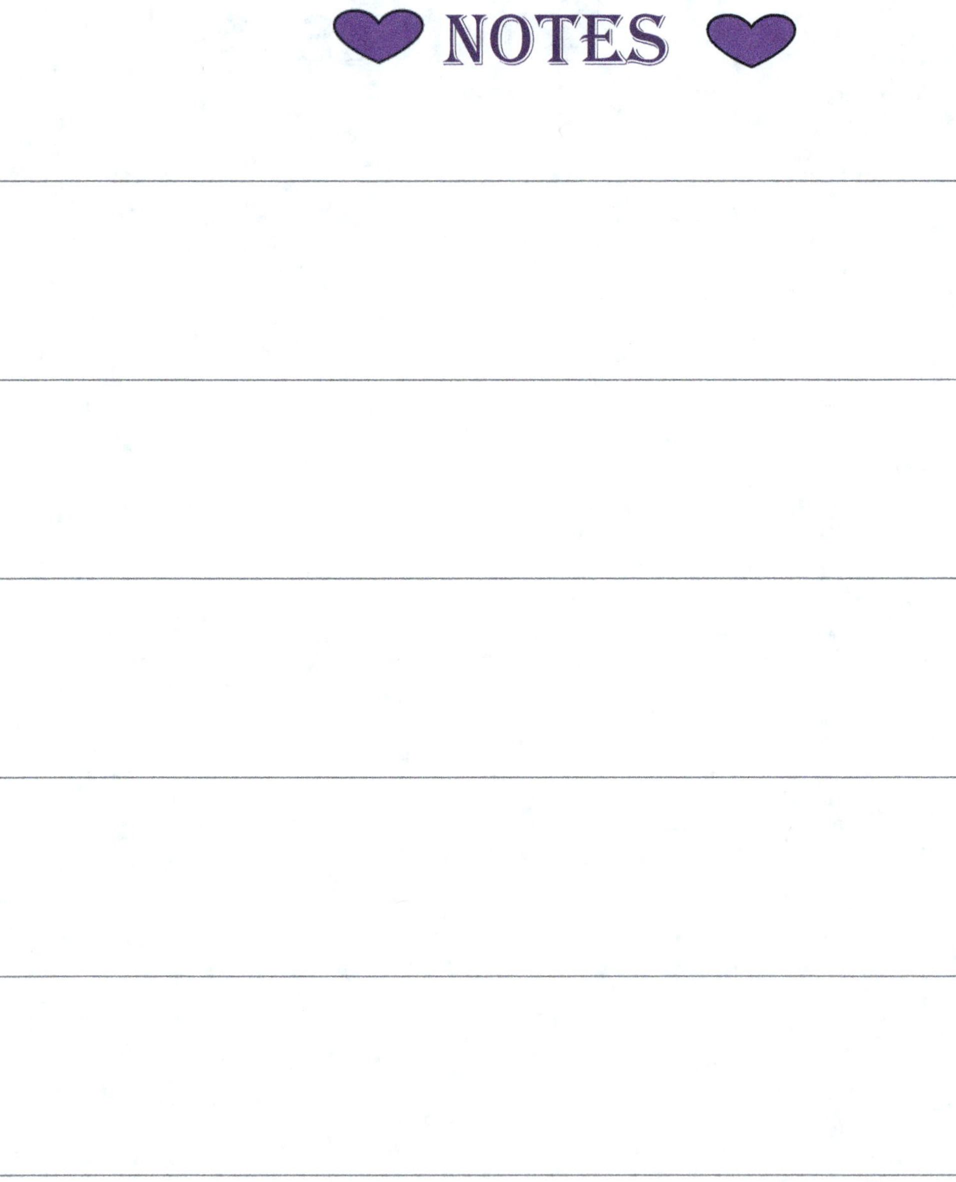

**Women, Permit Yourselves ~ To Be Well…**

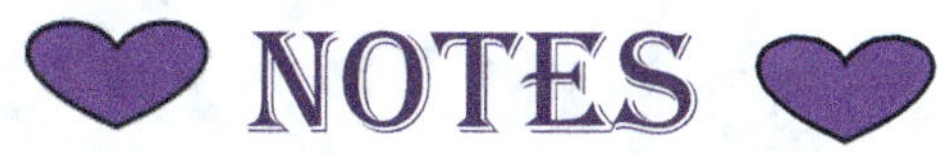

# NOTES

**Women, Permit Yourselves ~ To Be Well...**

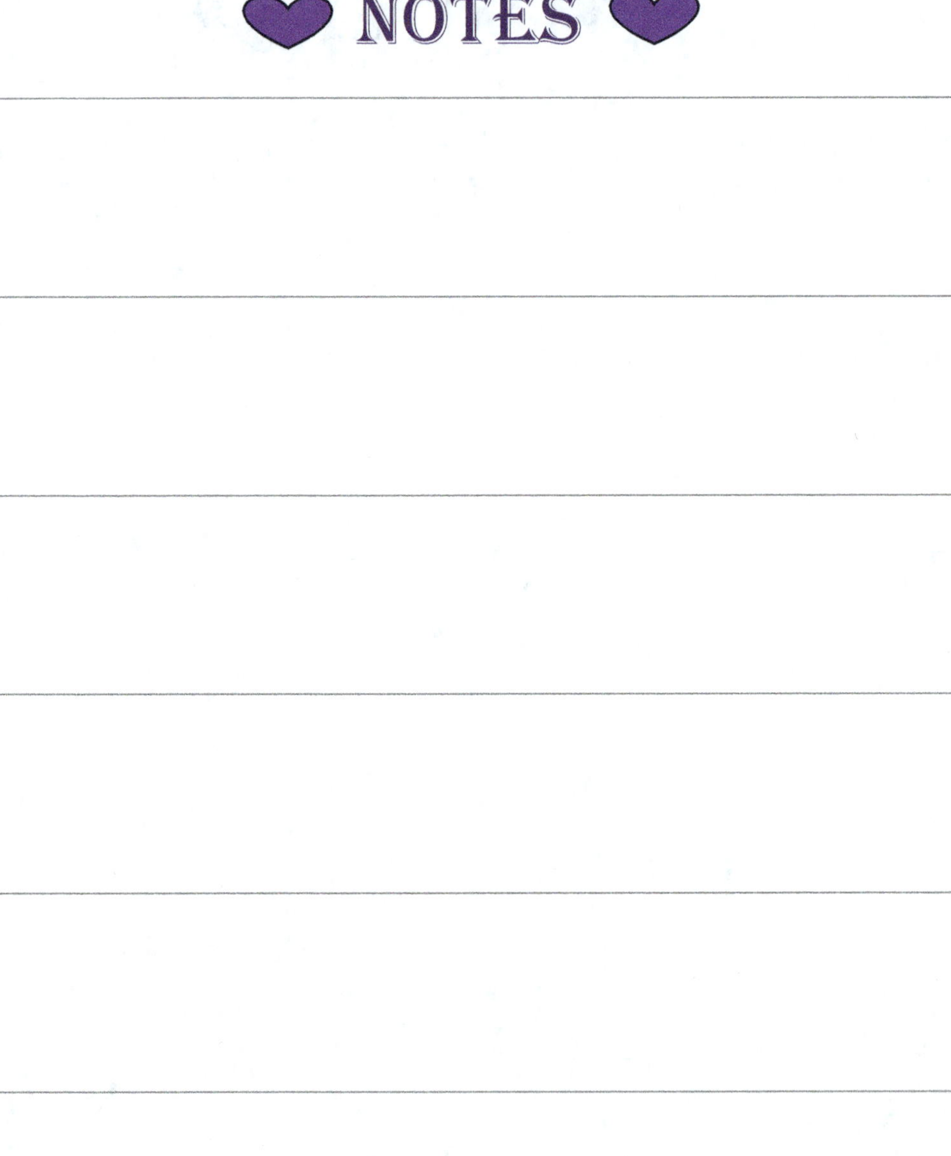

# 💜 NOTES 💜

**Women, Permit Yourselves ~ To Be Well…**

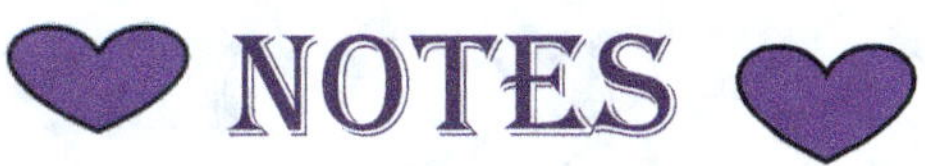

**Women, Permit Yourselves ~ To Be Well…**

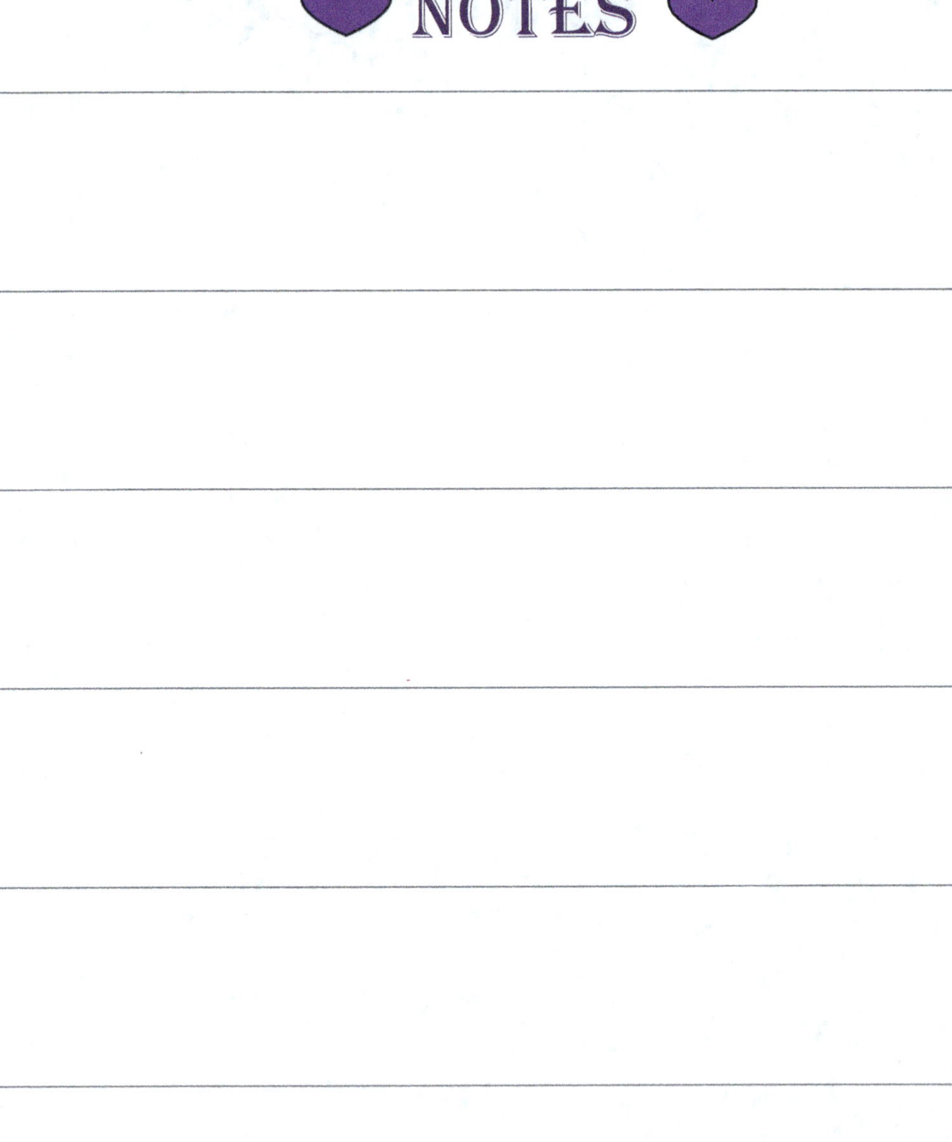

# ♥ NOTES ♥

**Women, Permit Yourselves ~ To Be Well…**

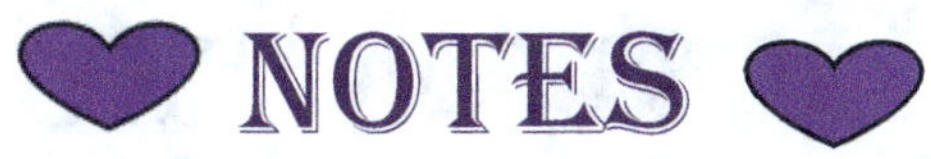

# ♥ NOTES ♥

**Women, Permit Yourselves ~ To Be Well…**

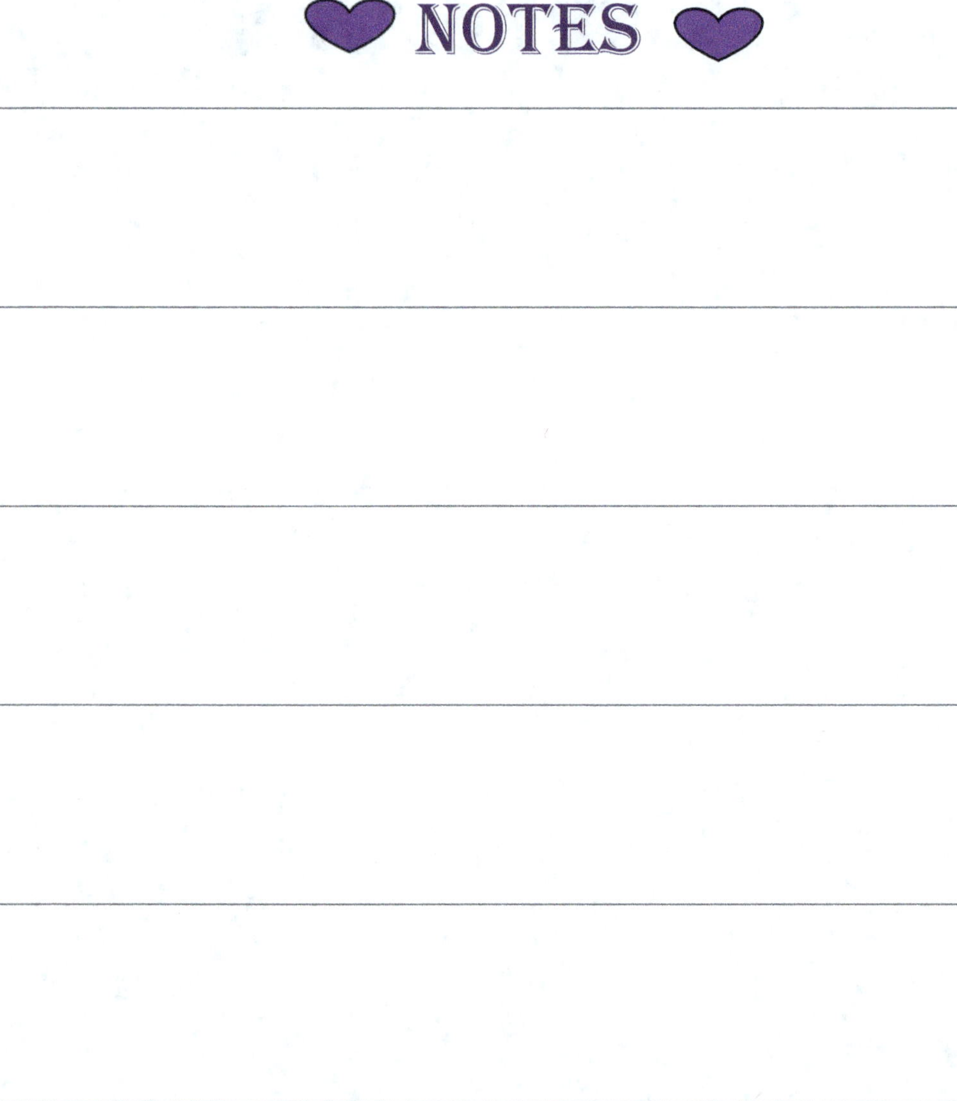

# ❤ NOTES ❤

---

**Women, Permit Yourselves ~ To Be Well...**

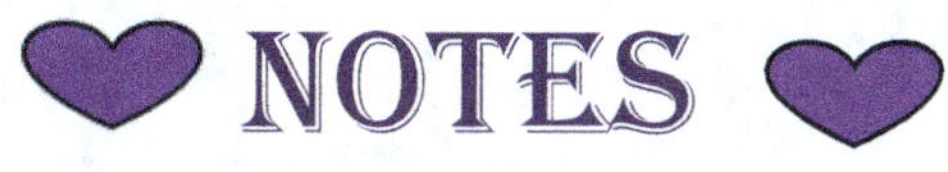

---